Secrets *of* Nursing

Ramona Radford

PublishAmerica
Baltimore

First printing

PublishAmerica has allowed this work to remain exactly as the author intended, verbatim, without editorial input.

ISBN: 1-60703-237-6
PUBLISHED BY PUBLISHAMERICA, LLLP
www.publishamerica.com
Baltimore

Printed in the United States of America

Secrets

of

Nursing

Nurses: who are they and what do they do? Have you ever been in the hospital or been in the presence of the nurse? She, or as you may now have he, is the kind-hearted person to see you prior to the doctor. I am the nurse. You know me. I smile and comfort you in your time of need while secretly holding back my own fears of what you may be facing. Prejudice to some and yet compassionate to others, we, the nurses of this healthcare profession, are used and abused professionally and publicly.

I am nearing my 25th year of nursing and have seen all that I care to see of it. No longer is nursing a way of giving back of yourself to the good of mankind. Rather nursing is the foothold of multi-billion-dollar businesses, privately owned and operated with no restrictions imposed other than state board of health commissions. Silence is eating me up inside. I must reveal to the world nursing as it is today, nursing 2000. At times I feel like a total trader to the profession that I'd loved so much. Are these nursing secrets new or age old since the beginning of nursing, since Florence Nightgale? The truth of the matter is you must stand for something or fall for anything.

Everyone may think of nursing as this pretty smiling face person, caring and loving and the job oh so rewarding, and easy. Well quite the contrary I am bitter at the way corporate heads are using the profession to hide behind. Nursing was a rewarding profession but now it has become an upmost chaotic. So called professional people in the field to save or restore lives together in partnership now tearing at each other's throats as to much overload of work demands have clouded our number one goal.

As time passes and the demand so greatly increases for nurses still on the rise, does any one wonder why this may be. Here are the downright disgusting truths of nursing and the decline of respect for it. Many are shock horrified of the content exposed within this book. Let not the professional people be frown upon but let's do investigate management and corporate heads.

Ask the question of nurse to patient ratio, or better yet doctor to patient ratio, and yet the people more directly in contact with the patient the CNA's to patient ratio, and see what numbers you get, I can tell you the numbers are astronomical and not because of a shortage of nurses but one of management to staff problem. Staffing agencies on the rise as a new one opens practical every day. Not every healthcare setting is poorly run and managed as I have seen some good ones but I must say that the bad ones outnumber the good.

To the family that have supported me and kept me from self destructive foolishness, and friends that have been there for me. I thank you.

Not so long ago, or so it may seem, in full eagerness to care for the sick and disabled I became a Medical Assistant. In 1980, I worked for varies doctor's offices as a Medical Assistant. The first job I had was working in a clinic seeing all kinds of people with general problems, not requiring hospitalization. My job was to screen the patient and do any lab draws the doctor would order the ones need to get results to treat that patient right away, some of the lab draws had to be sent off, as cultures take time to grow and results take longer to return.

Working in the lab was rewarding and fun as I've seen a crab, once a lady came into the clinic and gave a crab to the doctor, to prove to him that's what she really had, I took it placed on a microscope slide and found it to be quite colorful and interesting I understood now how it got its name for that's just what it looks like a crab.

The older gentleman that's kind of perverted likes to come in once a week for the B12 injections in the butt, tells me how he must get this injection as he is going to have a long weekend with his girlfriend, I detect a little sexual undertone as he looks back and smile at me. With the needle still in hand I give the injection as hard as I could to let him feel that I didn't appreciate his remarks.

Maybe one of the most interesting things thus far in the clinic a male transvasedic has come to the office for checkup? He/She only wanted to talk to the doctor so I got nothing from this person so I read the history report to my finding he had a surgery to invert the penis and now has a virgina oh how I wanted to assist in the exam but the doctor was the only one to see. I guess everything was going fine the doctor wrote a prescription for hormones and she left.

So young was I to have my first encounter with the ugly word prejudice the year was 1980. She walked into the office for lab test to be drawn, I greeted her took her back to the lab, sat up my equipment in my usual manner and out of her mouth came this roaring "you're not going to draw my blood" at first I thought maybe she was referring due to my age, not so, I overheard her tell the other nurse with no lab experience as myself she didn't want me because of the color of my skin.

As a valuable nurse to the doctor he defended my professionalism, and told the woman that she could take her business elsewhere if she didn't want me to draw her blood. Need I tell you I have never felt so much emotions whelming up inside, warm tears streaming down my face as though they were coming from the depths of my soul and yet I pulled myself together after hearing the doctors' words, and yes I drew her blood in silence. She thanked me for the gentleness she hadn't received before and left.

I respected the doctors I had worked with and vice versa. We worked and enjoyed being helpful this made the work a good place to be. It was a rather small office yet large in other ways that's what kept our business flowing with patients at a maximum on a daily bases. Soon the clinic closed I had worked there for more than 4 good years.

Moving forward with nursing still working in the clinical setting I entered into a specialist office. There we tested for allergies to the skin. Interesting field yet very boring putting drops of allergens on the back of patients waiting for results. Looking for the same rewarding feelings I had at the clinic I had worked at in the beginning of my career, I found a good office close to home with good benefits.

The office was located in a suite on the 5th or 6th floor of a larger building of doctors and specialist. The job requirements were more demanding as I schedule appointments kept the accounting books records of payment, back office work, and lab draws. But I didn't mind all the work load, because the doctor was a tall and handsome man and oh boy did he smell so good, and oh so married.

This didn't keep me from flirting with him. I wore tight reveling clothing, and had I continued working there, I would have slept with him; the doctor was also flirty doing the kinds of things that would put us into closeness with one other. His good looks and the smell of seductive cologne he wore, caused my short employment time and in search for another job. I liked being able to go from one job to the next at my leisure and to my appeal. Nursing had fed me and I wanted to see more.

Medical assisting was good start in the medical field for me, but I needed something else so I climbed the nursing ladder and became a CNA, certified nursing assistant in 1993. This job wasn't front or back office work rather that of patient care. CNA's work in hospitals and home care or Long Term Care facilities, better known as nursing homes. The pay was comparable and it seem like something I would like so I jump right in and went to a training class of basically common sense things like what to do and not do caring for elderly patients. Little did I know nursing asstisant job pay was comparable to a restaurant job pay, all the same I wanted to feel rewarding to someone else.

The first hands-on job or clinical was working with the elderly patients in the nursing home while being checked off for varies things like toileting, shaving the male patients, transferring, emptying a urinal, putting someone on the bed pan and making a bed correctly. Cleaning up solid elderly briefs was so disgusting that once while the class was in a male patient's room changing has solid brief, I ran from the room and just outside the room began gagging and earring.

How was I to do this job, it was like taking care of overgrown babies with giant diapers on. Then you look into those helpless eyes and think how you could not help them for they are so helpless. Many of them have such stories to tell about their lives and the places they had been now out of place awaiting to die. Family members come to visit on holidays and the facility tries to keep up with the festive decorating and dinner and all. Still there's no place like home.

I can remember working so hard in a eight hour shift there was nothing left of myself to give after leaving work and going home to my than small children. But the job was rewarding in a way that it paid the bills and you could work all the long hours that you could possible imagine, sometime working as many as sixteen plus hours a day. The patient load was unbelievable as we were responsible for getting the patients dress or undressed depending on the time of day it was and a patient load of 10 plus patients to 1 CNA.

Talk about back breaking work sure to kill anyone working as a CNA to long I thought. I can remember watching the nurses as they sit around eating lunch or talking on the phone, asking you to go help so and so and never lifting a finger to help you. I began to see the licensed nurses as my next climb up the nursing ladder. In 1996 I took my career path slow and continue to work as a CNA for about 2 years more while going to school first part time than full time for a LPN license. Now the nurse shortage has hit an all time high level of demand, why new people coming into the field want to feel like they are doing something rewarding or those whom have been in for a long time want out because of the stress of it all never the less a career in demand indeed.

Funny if no help showed up on the job and you did, the same amount of work was still required of you only more of it, and this usually happened just about pay day. The staff is most likely to call in sick during pay days and weekends, some places changed pay day from weekend to during the week pay periods. The older worker would be the loyal ones to come in, but more likely to call off for sickness, in contrary the younger staff would call off for practical everything.

Some of the food that the dietary people cooked was the same old boring stuff day after day. Most of the patients were thin from not eating for various reasons but more so because of the food preparations. I really believed that by becoming a nurse I could make a difference in someone life, but how? I didn't know I just knew that I didn't want to become some old woman with gray hair and a bad back with bad feet still working as a CNA.

I couldn't complain I had worked enough hours brought a new car and had enough money to put the down payment for a home. Yes I brought a home on CNA money I had worked long and hard never did I enjoy my home as most of the time I was sleeping or getting up to go back to work. This was a vicious cycle day in day out but the corporate people didn't mind they just wanted a warm body ready to do the impossible.

This is how a typical shift assignment would start. You begin by showing up seeing how many workers are there and split up the patients. The night shift was responsible for getting people up and on nights they would have less CNA due to the lack of activities going on and oh yes everyone is asleep. During this time I called it the check and change time supposedly everyone had to be turned every 2 hours and changed if necessary, if you are working shorthanded that 2 hours may turn into 4 to 6 hours or just before leaving an 8 to 12 hour shift so not to make anyone angry.

Have you ever tried to sitting or lying in one position for a long period of time say 2 hours or more? I can tell you it's not easy feeling all the pressure on one area it's downright hard to do, your body starts to tingle in pain in the area of the most pressure sending signals to the brain saying move but you can't and the pain intensifies to the point of becoming numb. It's no wonder that more than half the people there have the most hideous wounds called pressure ulcers those that can't turn themselves or those that are incontinent with fire red bottoms worst than a baby's bottom with diaper rash. Now you have 2 in 1 problems the incontinent patient with a pressure ulcer equals infection.

On the night shift we wouldn't tell the patient what we were doing just go in turn on the lights and begin doing our job. We would flip you bottom side up check you slid a pad under your bottom along with brief toss you from side to side assuring the fit and flip you to the opposite side you where laying on. If it was your day for a shower you would get a shower between midnight and 3 a.m. because at 3 a.m. everyone is preparing to get dress for the morning, and remember we had to get up as many as 6 to 10 people, the morning people had to get up the ones still in bed serve trays and feed people.

People laying in bed were awaken to sometimes wet cold spray on their bottoms the stuff used to clean incontinence, or wet cold wash clothes. Some of the people resistant, angry, and fighting why wouldn't you if someone enter your room without saying a word flip on all the lights in the room throw back the covers flip you over and rip the bed pad from underneath you replace it with two or more pads to make the bed check go a little faster the next time around. There was no pride left for all that went away after walking through the front doors. Some would complain to the family but nothing was done to change what would happen day in and day out.

Let's see what happens on day shift, more workers would show up to work days because this is when you have the corporate heads in for a few hours walking around to see what kind of head count is there. Head count of patients and money, were their only concern, not if the patient was receiving good care or how many patient per caregiver ratio. No census up or down was their concern. I thought to myself how could they be so blind to the way the place is run, and how could state come in and not see the mess these people were in.

After getting up the few people still left down in bed the day shift CNA would hurry those who could feed themselves to one dining room while those that had to be fed to another room. The morning meal usual came between 7:30 a.m. and 8:00 a.m. and to complete everyone was about 9:30, 10:00 then the routine would be lay them down till lunch. Most of the time they wouldn't be laid down or would stay up with the same brief put on at 3:00 a.m., and oh how the place smelled of urine that same brief until time for the next shift or just prior to getting off.

Second shift no better than the one before they come in and some people would be in the wheel chair drenched with urine or feces or laying in bed with it. When you walk into a long term care facility and the first thing you smell is the stench you better believe it's from the lack of care, stemming from the lack of help. Each shift is responsible for a certain amount of showers per day so between the meals and laying down showers are to be done; everything is a hurry, hurry, and rush.

Skin tears and falls are on the raise some reported and others not reported. The bigger the facility the worst the help in it is. Now second shift has completed an evening meal which started at 5:00 p.m. lasting for approximately 2 hours, showers and putting to bed for the night has started. Hygiene is of least important until the stench is offensive to everyone around the patient than heads start turning and people want something done now. Teeth and hair and skin are hardly of any importance as the patients teeth began rotting out or become loose and fall out while eating, hair is combed as needed, and the skin is never moisten so it becomes dry cracked and flaking, also nails are thick long dirty and lastly ears thick with wax that ear drops have to put in to loosen up wax buildup than irrigated after one week.

It matters not what one person does to try to help the patients if everyone is not doing their part, this job will break the best hearted person down to his knees and will give in to the I don't care syndrome.

You begin to wonder who cares the management don't care and so why should you. But having a compassionate heart for the good of others keeps you from conforming to the norm. Second shift people lay the people down for the night shift to come in and continue with care. By about 7:30, 8:00 p.m.

everyone is in bed for the night. Those people who are diabetic are supposing to get snacks don't and in the morning blood glucose levels are low or bottoming out. Patients going to the hospital and being diagnosis with dehydration why because the very least of things like water is not offered not within reach or not easily accessible. CNA's are responsible for getting water pitchers filled with fresh water and or ice every shift, but this rarely gets done but possibly once a shift. Some patients never drink but the small amounts of water given by the nurse to take a pill.

The night shift or 3rd.shift get shift differational why, I think because of the hour at night it becomes extremely hard to stay awake and so most of the staff do sleep some part of the night. During the night shift patients are neglected the most. Call lights go unanswered; those that are incontinent stay that way for several hours until the last minute of the shift. Water pitcher goes without being filled UTI frequently seen in the elderly patients leading to major chemical imbalances and eventual death left undiagnosed and untreated.

QMA's, or qualified medicine assistants, LPN's, licensed practical nurses, and 1 to 2 RN's, registered nurses, and the most valued person working the CNA's, certified nursing assistants, are the people to run the long term care facilities. On any given day you will find one RN in the building covering some state regulatory, but mostly QMA's and LPN's work along side of the CNA to meet the needs of the patients. The Q as they are called can only pass meds. All other nursing must come from the LPN, or RN. Things like access the patient for vitals and any blood monitoring equipment for blood sugar levels, any Gastro feeding tubes, and all injections must have a nurse perform.

The help that each of the nursing staff gives is vital to the care and needs of the patients they must work together or fall apart. Helpful to some extent is the QMA but at times you all most want to just do the entire job yourself because half the job of the nurse gets done and the nurse is left to do what the Q can't do. I was placed on a 60 plus patient hall with 2 Q and I worked harder working between the 2 than just taking one cart and passing meds to 30 patient. That was the usually happening when the long term care facility was running short of help. The Q's would work as needed, sometimes working as CNA's as that is what they came from prior to learning how to pass meds.

Let's not forget the CNA's they are the hardest working people, I know cause I've been there done that. You have to have some compassionate for humanity, because changing soiled adults of urine and feces is not an easy job. In fact once while in training for a CNA I had to run out of a patient's room erring as the smell of fecal matter had engulfed me, I wondered than could I do this job. I saw my other classmates performing the job of clean up this patient with ease, as if they did smell a thing.

LPN's and RN's work closely together for the education level is relatively connected; the RN's having more clinical time than that of the LPN. Each of these nurses can take critical orders from the doctor and transpose them to physician order sheets if the doctor has to call in orders, so that the pharmacy will fill that order and wait for a doctor's signature later. Some new RN's feel as though school has made them better than the rest of the nursing staff having that title but what really matters is the experience. I have had to teach some of the RN's coming out of school simple things like how to cath a patient.

Here is the usual routine in most long term care facilities, and like restaurants business if you have seen one you seen them all. The only thing different is the faces of the people you take care of. Consequential the residents that live there are the ones to suffer from the capitalization of big corporate business making billions of dollars from the poor and shut out.

Treatment of wounds are done per shift with some of the larger dressing changes left for the night shift nurse as she/he has the least of work to do. The night nurse is overloaded with double the residents than any other shift for the least amount of activity is going on. She also gets a bigger shift differential for her efforts to stay awake during these hours of sleep for most people. I can tell you I have work every shift and the night shift is the worst shift for after working it you feel like a zombie.

Doctors in long term care also become overwhelm with the patient load well over 100 patients per doctor. I often wonder how the doctor can see so many patients and have outside patients somewhere else and keep all patient cases straight? Daily the picture becomes clearer that these once productive people of society no longer are useful but are now a burden to society and family. What happen to family values and traditions, when there weren't any nursing home facilities?

My experience as a nurse in the hospital was a totally new environment with all kinds of situations. The nurse on days has the most amount of workload running frantic to meet all the needs of the doctor, social worker and any therapy people that might need to see that patient. The patient ratio being 5 to 1 and sometimes 5 patients could be a bit much. Second shifts are pretty much the same as day shift and nights still the same not like your typical long term care nurse patient ratio on nights at maximum 1 to 7 or 8 depending on the acuity level.

When I speak on acuity level is the level of care the patient might need IV's, a drop in vital signs that have to be monitor or just in general sick and needing much attention. Some of the hospital have come up with 12 hour shifts were as a nurse has the option of working 3 shifts day or night shift, usually 3 days on 4 days off, to have the benefit of being off for more days. But with all the time the nurse has off she feels complied to work extra shift or two or three in a work week.

Over worked nurse make costly mistakes some reported others covered up as the nurse would not dare show incompetence. She has to live up to her title of knowing all unblemished from making an error those errors that are reported everyone would know about it, she is looked upon as incompetent, and written up to be placed in her personal records. How safe is the person taking care of you or your loved one after working 12 hour shifts on a week to week bases? Has the increasing economy demand caused us to become careless, and heartless? Doctors do the same, long hours and in an abundant of patients they hardly knew, they would come in to check on the patient and have not a clue about them other than what the nurse can tell them.

Medication overload and medication interaction has always fascinated me the people in the long term care facilities that would take in excess of 10 plus medications a day where as the people in the hospital took very few but those in the hospital would receive in excess of 2 to 3 different antibiotics nearly back to back. It become apparent that maybe the IV solutions should just be mixed in one and given together but what did I know I was only the nurse.

A lot of infidelity is seen on the job this per domically female work environment with males dominating as doctors is it any wonder why this shouldn't happen. So many lies told and secrets in the air about the nursing staff and doctors who loved this one and that one. You could write the next soap opera based on the daily events in the hospital.

Doctors, nurses and other healthcare professional are suppose to be a team working together to help the patient but doctors seem to take their title a little far belittle the nurse talking to them harsh and with short tempers, demanding and just downright nasty. As though nurses were restaurant hostess, and other times when you had to call the doctor on the phone at night some of them would listen and say o.k. and hang the phone up on you so hard you felt it on the other end. If not for the so called little people under the doctor once again the doctor would not have a clue of what's going on with the patient.

Working in the hospital was exciting for the most part seeing different people all the time with all kinds of illness. But what I didn't like is the covering up of errors. Things like giving the wrong medication or the wrong antibiotic to the wrong patient. I still say that overworked healthcare professional is a danger to everyone. Some errors are made due to nurses using drugs either from taking the patient's or from home.

A vicious hate among two RN charge nurses nearly cost a man his life. The night charge nurse sits up the day charge nurse by putting a license nurse on the floor with high acuity, IV's and ventilators a floor that the license nurse is unfamiliar with. The night nurse makes assignments out for the following shift she knew very well that the license nurse stay away from this floor because she had no experience and everyone else knew not to assign her to this unit. Out of hate for one another the day charge nurse forces the nurse to stay in spite of her reluctance she was going to work on all the units not just the rehab. As the day goes on the license nurse asks for help from the charge nurse making this day a living hell for the charge this was planned from the night charge nurse to happen. The doctor writes an order to give the license nurse's patient an antacid medicine the patient was getting through his gastric tubes orders are to give IV. The license nurse questions the doctor he in turn tells her "I ordered that way, that's what I want" so the license nurse never giving any meds through the IV goes to the refrigerator takes out the man's antacid and draws it up in a syringe. The license nurse starts to push the medicine and finds it too thick to push so she thins it by adding water to the solution. The only thing that saved the man's life is that myself and the Respiratory Therapist was sitting watching the Telemetry strips and notice the patient going into distress, at the time the Respiratory Therapist and I enter the room to find the nurse pushing the solution in the IV. The patient survived after a code blue distress alarm was sent out.

The day charge nurse quit the night one followed the same and quit also. Talk about nasty it happens more times than not and the patients are the ones to suffer.

The stress from nursing causes some nurses to find other avenues to cope be it stimulants, antidepressants or just plain old alcohol. The nurses as well as the doctors too get pump up for the day with their coffee mugs filled with alcohol you can smell on their breaths, some try to cover up with gum but it doesn't always help. Their eyes and skin tell the truth but no one says anything, as if this was to protect the healthcare profession creditability. I can remember telling the Director of Nursing or the DON as she is called and the person continue to work there under those conditions.

Stealing of narcotic drugs from the patient is seen more and more, it has become a common way that a nurse can keep up a habit of drug abuse. I have seen many nurses in handcuffs being escorted out of the building. What an embarrassment to themselves and the nursing profession to have happen. Some nurses take lunch breaks go out of building or not, do the drugs prescribed to their patient come back and continue taking care of patients. There are others that steal the drugs not to use but to sale. It's like putting an alcoholic behind a bar and telling them not to drink, same with nursing professionals with a drug abuse problem and that goes for young and old alike. I have seen my co-worker in the bathroom at work with a needle stuck in his arm trying to get high at work passed out in the bathroom near death once an employee now becoming the patient.

A well known surgeon during the day and at night out smoking crack cocaine prior to going to work the next morning, spending money with nurses that will protect his surgeon life during the day. Who better than someone in the healthcare to keep matters quite, he would spend as much needed to have a good time but sometime early morning he'd sleep and off to work he'd go. Once he even offered a substantial amount of money to see two nurses having sex as he said the cocaine desensitize him. I wanted to report him but felt like I would be betraying the healthcare profession. Another time a nurse who faithfully came in to work high on something was found in one of the empty rooms on the floor in a patient's room, so high she didn't know where she was. She had all the signs of substance abuse and yet the hospital continues to allow the nurse to work because she was an RN and needed for a charge nurse.

Nursing is a stressful job with a huge amount of responsibility with little recognition for the efforts. Nurses are compassionate people with large hearts being misused by corporate and private own healthcare businesses. They have made the nurses envy one another and brought about hatred among them, by making nurses use their titles to confess that RN's are better than LPN's or CNA titles whereby pushing the LPN's out of the hospitals and into long term care facilities. Still needing CNA's to help as someone has to clean up the mess how awful because it's everyone's responsibility to help.

I personally knew a nurse whose husband and her both doing and saleing drugs were at the hospital where I was working the husband in serious condition on his death bed speak. The wife his nurse ask that none of us nurses working had to do any of his care because she was going to take care of him herself and I thought well this is her husband so why not let her do for him. Later I realize she was stealing the drugs we brought in to him or so we suspected her of doing, as his condition worsen, he was put on hospice and an IV line was started. The drug of choose being Dilaudid on a continuous pump and on demand. He was too weak to push the demand button so his wife did the pushing for him and when it was empty the staff nurses would put in a new cassette. Somehow towards the end of his life the wife crafted a way to steal the entire remending narcotic out of the cassette. Upon his death the IV was stop and the usual is for two nurses to witness the destruction or waste of the remaining drug, but when we beginning to destroy the drug we noticed there was none there.

There was an investategation and all of the nurses who had any kind of dealing with this patient were a suspect of the missing drug. Through careful logging of the uses of the oncoming and outgoing nurses it was pin point to just at the time of death that the drug came up. The officers found that a pin point puncture was made probably that of a needle and the drug was withdrawn out. I immediately figured out that the wife had crafted this ideal and a brilliant one at that who would have even thought of such a thing. As time passed I hadn't seen much of this nurse until one day while working for the staffing agency I ran into her and that feeling of I know what you done came over me. I never told anyone what I knew but she knew that I knew what she had done. She had put everyone of the nurses in the crime light for what she had done. Many nurses today have problems of drug abuse and can't be around narcotic drugs, or not allowed to handle narcotic but can pass non-narcotic drugs to patients, mandated through a nursing rehabilitation program. So sad to see a nurse say I can't handle narcotic but can you pass my narcotic to my patient for me, contrary to this nurse, another nurse, in the middle of shift is being lead out of the building in hand cuffs by the police. There have been reports of nurses taking old used Fentanyl patches off patients that have worned them for 3 days and taking the residue medicine out of the patch by using a needle to extract the residue out and using it. This alarmed me why would anyone use something that was already used up for 3 days now? I examined the patches we threw away and sure as day it showed residue meds still in the clear patches used. Some places like hospital required nurses to destroy the patches with a second nurse to witness the destruction. Wow there is nothing that the drug seeking person wouldn't craft up.

A personal associate of mine, due to a battery charge lost her healthcare license. She assumed another friend's license and the two of them shared the same name and worked in separated places. Under the license they filed taxes together, and the taxes where split. This went on for some time and then the one without the license stopped working in the healthcare profession. I never wanted to know any details. Another nurse busted for drug use loses her license still working in nursing under someone else license. I had worked with this nurse in a hospital knew her, and her children; she was once called under one name prior to her departure, now working under an assumed name. While working through the agency ran into her coming on shift she was to be my relief the staff member spoke to her not the name I knew, and at that moment our eyes met and she knew that I knew that the name was not her own. Her eyes seem to silently beg me not to say anything and I didn't.

Narcotics are counted after each shift by the oncoming nurse the outgoing nurse reads off the listed number of remaining count and both agree to sign off the corrected amount. Being crafted the outgoing nurse would say the correct count but not have the written correct count so as the outgoing nurse read off the number the ongoing nurse had better look on the pages also. Other crafted things were done with the narcotics things like taking a bottle of morphine liquid and replace some or all with cough syrup. A patient once was receiving morphine liquid for his pain the patient was not getting the desired affect the doctor had intended for him to get so the doctor switched over to something else stronger, little did anyone know the morphine had been replaced with cough syrup until the time of destroying it and this patient suffered severe pain all to the hands of a not so caring nurse.

Long term care nursing take on a whole new world of nursing and just like those things that happen in the hospital setting like stealing of drugs and infidelity go on, the same things happen here stealing of drugs are on the higher rate. My first impression of the building after being hired on as a nurse was good. I toured the building along with the others that had been hired and now on orientation. The tour began with the very nice air conditioned lobby full of nice furniture tress, plants, paintings, and such. Then on to the rehab department with its array of fitness equipment, I'm impressed.

Next on the tour we went behind the scenes to the units as they were called, it was little stepping out of heaven into hell. First was the stench of urine and feces aroma filling the air so forcing one to want to hold your breath for fear of earring. The old familiarity came back to me but now I was the nurse and not the CNA. I went into the nursing home, not willingly, now that the hospital was no longer utilizing LPN's in the fullest capacity as nurse we were taught to be.

The facility vowed in its admission statement to provide a safe, clean, comfortable, and homelike environment, allowing the resident to use his or her personal belongings to the extent as possible. Some of these things were provided but not all, most of the time the place reek of urine and bowel. Homelike possible there were cats roaming and birds in their cages fling around. Personal belongings were no longer personal but community property when the CAN"s couldn't find what was needed to complete the patient that they would be with like borrowing hygiene products, brushes or combs, that sort of things. Also in the statement housekeeping and maintenance services necessary to maintain a sanitary, orderly, and comfortable interior would be provided. Housekeeping was provided while the management was there and anytime state would be coming to do the annual walk through. Some facilities use hopers to clean solid linen prior to washing it, no one wanted to use the hopers to hose the really solid BM linen so most of the bad linen went to garbage. Other things in the mission statement to have a clean bed and bath linens that are in good condition that usually happen. Private closet space in each resident room with clothes racks and shelves accessible to the resident if available you had a private closet.

Adequate and comfortable lighting levels in all areas, usually not all areas in all places.

So many restrictions being enforced now upon the LPN's that they couldn't do much of any nursing without the RN signature behind each of your nursing assessments and they never accessed the patient they patient of their own so they just signed next to your signature going along with corporate decisions. There was a lot of hate in the air you could cut it with a knife. You never knew when someone was going to set you up for failure. Corporate also decided that if the RN was doing so much work for the LPN then she shouldn't have but a maximum of 2 patients and the LPN would get 6 to 7 patients so the RN could set around and watch you run yourself in the ground working. Many times I needed help and would ask the RN for help they would get upset, what a horrible thing these corporate people had done to nursing.

Once there was a time when 2 RN's were sitting at the table received a call, about one of my patients on telemetry heart rate had dropped down in the 40tys. And because I wasn't there to take the call, they negated to come find me to let me know this. A CNA came to me about the matter and informed me of what she had overheard the 2 of them plotting not to tell me. I thought to myself how curial can you get and that was the last straw for me my patient's life was in jeopardy all because corporate had decided to make one nurse superior to the other.

Getting back to my new job as the nursing home nurse, I was very much welcomed as a nurse and paid a good salary that was higher than or comparable to my hospital pay. I wanted to make a difference from what I had seen before working in the nursing home. Soon after working there I found it to be just what I had seen only worst. The nurses overworked with 30 plus patients or residents as they were called. The CNA's responsible for 15 plus residents, each resident needier than the other.

Being responsible for so many patients one is sure to make fail able errors in medication and miss treatments, orders from the doctor of a medication change that don't get taken off in a timely manner. The things of the most importance were unable to be finished due to the overwhelming work load expected of you. The responsibilities included patient follow ups, taking off orders from the doctors, doing treatments to wounds and buttock creams which almost everyone received because of incontinence episodes, skin assessments, vital signs once a month, pertinent charting on incidence or falls, and last the end of the month change over the rewrites as they are called where something always got missed putting the old orders and new ones on the new medication books because it took more than one nurse to do the end of the month rewrites.

Some patients still received medications that where discontinued and other medications that where suppose to be continued where discontinued what a mess. At the end of every month the rewrites had to be done and as sure as they were done something was sure to be missed as everyone had a hand in doing rewrites. Rewrites are medication sheets from the previous month with all the added changes in medication. This was a must to do along with the other assignment of being the nurse. So each shift the nurse would do so many charts until the entire unit was completed. The corporate people would be seen just prior to state coming in for their annual inspections they would tell management people how to clean up house to look the way it should when state wasn't there, that would keep nosey inspectors from prying too far. And so it was much like cleaning house prior to awaiting company at your own home, everyone would clean up the units and extra help was allowed on the floors, it's sad that inspections where the only time extra help would be called.

Consider the everyday life of each person as I reveal the residents of the units to whom I have worked with no names to protect confidentiality. I have kept all my assignments and remember each patient as each is unique in their own way. With the ratios of staff to patients being so high some patients that were less alert meds or treatments were either omitted or given all at once if there weren't any repeat meds. Understand, than, those patients that were alert were usually the ones to get meds and treatments accordingly as ordered as they knew what they were due and what times. If the patients were a constant complainer they would receive some type of as needed med, or prn as it is called whether it was their own or narcotic drugs prescribed for someone else were given to quite the patient. When medications wouldn't help and the patient was becoming more irritating to the nurse or the CNA the call would be taken away. In short those that could not do for themselves were grossly negated clearly this was wrong but in light of the enormous amount of work these were the least recognized.

Patients on hospice usually comfort measures only were given copious amounts of narcotics to keep the patient sedated meaning pain free, the drug of chooses being IV push morphine. This drug would be ordered to be pushed every one to two hours, as needed for pain, through intravenous catheter inserted to keep the vain open to push medicines and antibiotic through. Nurses who have an addiction would steal the morphine from the patient suspecting that the patient wasn't in pain because the drug was ordered to be given on an hourly bases, some of the morphine would be given some taken and no one would be the wiser. Once while taking a break the charge nurse signed out a narcotic intended for my patient, but when I returned the patient stated she didn't receive it who should you believe nurse, or patient.?

Once there was an older nurse no one would have ever suspected of stealing narcotics busted caught in the act of stealing narcotics. She'd come into work at night tried all the time, she told us her son wouldn't allow her to sleep. I taught she had a young son under the age of 10 or so, but when I asked her she said he was 20 years old I also asked her why she allowed him to treat her like that when he needed to be put out of the house on his butt. The son paid no bills had no job and she would be on the phone most of the time that she was at work talking to him on the phone. So boldly and oddly I gave the nurse a piece of my mind, she told me I wouldn't understand he was sickly. This nurse came to work with bandages on every finger her arms wrapped up told us that she had burned herself on the stove, and still little did anyone know her son was abusing her and forcing her to steal drugs, until the day she got busted stealing narcotics and confessed her guilt.

A bad experience of mine came as I worked for an agency went to a nursing home to work in a pretty well to do place on the outside, but like most others I'd worked for the staffing was not available for the work load. It was an even shift I'd agreed to work as I walked up to the nursing station and presented myself the nurse on duty, a staff nurse seem to be in a hurry to leave give me a quick report on the two halls of patients that went like this: patient #1 takes meds crushed, this one whole meds, this one crushed in applesauce, and so on till the list was finished and by the way so and so has a temp., and here's a list of numbers in case you need to call someone, that was the usual report given to the agency nurse as if that was the most important. I began my shift looking through the med book for and diabetics I had to give insulin to or check blood levels on, when one of the CNA came to me in a frantic and told me that the patient was acting different today usually gets up for meals, now unable to get up. I left my work to assess the situation to find the person in bed with an inverted leg that look like the hip was bulging out and the lower part of the leg turned inward. Immediately I called all the necessary heads, and MD. Receive orders to send out. It was done paperwork done and patient gone, what struck me was the CNA's alarmed face made we suspect that she had tried to get the patient up alone, without proper equipment or help from someone else, and dropped the patient onto the floor and then put the patient back to bed. I will never know how it happened just glad to know I was able to help.

Working through the agency I have found myself looking at outdated pictures of nursing home residents and mistakenly given the wrong patient the wrong medication or the patient with dementia answers to the roommates name and gets the wrong meds. I Thank God I haven't seriously harmed anyone but did I tell anyone to know if in fact the med would interact no I just said nothing, and did my own evaluation. CNA's are usually helpful pointing out the resident to you; until they see that you're from the agency that's when everyone disappears and you can't find them for hours everyone just seem to take break at once without telling you. Everyone that I have had encounters with while working for the agency, in the long term care facilities or hospitals work on staff because they don't want to risk the chance of being cancelled from a shift which would cost them money. So staff people have all kinds of beef with the management from the pay to the work yet they continue to work there, under unfavorable conditions. Who reaps the abuse and neglect none other than the patients.

Unit 1A as I shall call it has two sides each side having more than 30 patients, very few independent residents many well in advanced total care residents. As I start down the hall of 1A there are 2 residents of the same capacity both having gastrointestinal feeding tubes with a large bag of feeding going at a rate the dietician has prescribed? In the first bed a woman that has had a severe stroke and cannot talk but the eyes follow you as you come into the room and start any kind of procedure with her, you can tell that she is in there but her entire body can't move. She lays in her own waste until someone comes in to change her, flies land on her face but she can't swat them away she release a tear from her eyes in the still of quietness. The second bed the woman is very much contracted but moves upper body tries to pull out her gastrointestinal feeding tube she is trapped inside and tries to stop any care that would prolong her life but without success, these two women await death while the families of the two come to look on the face of this lifeless shell. Negated you bet, if these women were more than likely would not receive the meds and or treatment because these women aren't considered a priority, and where are they going anyhow. Little output from them due a lack of water flushes into the gastro feeding tube, a simple process to do but with all the other patient demand not enough time to set there and put water down the tube and wait for it to go down cost you time, time you didn't have to waste on one patient.

Next is a retired nurse and her roommate, the nurse having Parkinson disease and memory lost falls out of bed and has to have a alarm on the bed and chair at all times. The roommate alert and orientated looks on in despair as she sees her roommate decoration daily. Both of these ladies on medications for pain and anxiety even when there is no evidence of that being diagnosed more than 50% of patients have this diagnosis. But in the nursing facility everyone is on some kind of pain and anxiety medicine. I tried to do my best and be on top of all things but even the best become wary and dismay I was guilty of negate.

Once on this unit I had a patient to fall on the floor and the policy states that vital signs had to be done every 15 minutes for 1 hour than every 30 minutes for the next 2 hours than every 8 hours for 72 hours. Trying to be the best nurse that I could be I began to do the vitals and found that the other 30 plus patients were being negated, I stopped to help the other patients and was only able to get a few vitals throughout the shift. The next day the unit manager was telling me that there were some holes in my paper work and they needed to be filled in I explained to her that I was unable to get the vital signs according to the policy she looked at me and winked her eye as she whispered just put in something everybody does. As I began to write down the vitals I hadn't gotten I was thinking to myself she just gave me the O.K. to lie, I also thought that if anything should happen to my patient the corporate people would stand clean and my name, signature on paperwork falsely stating things I hadn't done and who would be the blame should this matter gone to court, as some cases do.

I continued on working there, humbling myself to the norm at this facility not to make waves but my heart was troubled. I committed myself to work there and with no other employment insight for the LPN that I am, nursing homes seemed all that I could get, or work agency and get work here and there. Even when there weren't any occurrences like falls there was always that one person or persons sick requiring more time than you could give, so to provide care to the most people doing the least amount of harm those that could talk and were alert received their meds, and those who couldn't did not sad to say. When I approach the management about the problem of too much work they told me that this is the way it is and I had better get used to it if I was going to work in the nursing home. I thought to myself Lord please let me not have to go to a nursing home myself or my family.

Usually there was more incidence of falls and follow-ups that needed to be done in one shift than not. When you have more than one your day is consumed with work that is supposed to be finished at the end of the shift. Sometimes I would find myself not taking a break for anything not even to use the bathroom. Then you have family members calling to check on the patients you would need to stop what you are doing and answer questions or pull the charts to find the answer. Doctors didn't make matters better leaving tons of now orders that needed to be taken off. Some days, because the medication were so routine, I would give them by memory those people that I knew medicines that way I could cut down on having to look in the med book to see what the patient needed and there were times those medicine would have been changed in dosages or cut out altogether. The times would be off but at least they got there meds not at the right times but the med book would be signed out as so whether they had received their meds or not. But book holes were counted as unacceptable so many times blood pressures and other vital signs were falsified according to allowable time. The CNA books were also falsified no one had time to see what the patient was doing in the past and what he was doing at present so you just followed along with what was written days prior this made charting much easier for staffing, new staff members and agency people so that no holes were found.

Isolation rooms were shared I never understood the meaning of isolation in the nursing home when the room had two residents in it. In the hospital isolation was just that one person in the room alone, now the nursing home was telling me that it was o.k. for two people to be in the isolation room together. One patient infected the other not. The spread of disease is rapid in the nursing homes, the staff is trying to get through a shift and hand washing between patients is the least of priority. I found myself using the hand sanitizer in place of washing or not, as I was busy trying to get to all my assigned patients and that was a lot. I've seen some of the staffing use a bare hand, no gloved, to wash a patient's soiled bottom. Then the doctor to figure out the spread of infection runs so rapid. Even some procedures are performed with little precautions.

The next set of ladies, one with a bed alarm sensor to alarm when the patient has attempted to get up without assistance, the other a foreign woman, both incontinent and get up to go to the dining room for meals. Bed alarms were misused as the CNA's would turn them off if the patients was getting up to much and there again taking up to much time on one patient, so the patient usually fell on the floor and the incident was made up the alarm malfunctioned. The foreign woman doesn't seem to mind her roommates alarm going off nor does she seem to care about the constant yelling out. One of the woman have to be fed and that is part of the nurse's responsibility because the CNA's take a many of the feed patients to feeding room and the rest of the patients on the floor were the nurses' to feed.

There are private rooms and semiprivate rooms, whereas most of the rooms are semi-private with two patient accommodations this room can accommodate two but is occupied by one person. She gets around in her mobilized chair and requires minimum assistance transferring just stand by assist of one staff member, she is quit demanding and takes a lot of time to put her just right in order that she likes when her call light goes off it goes unanswered for long periods of time because there isn't enough help to help her with her needs. So alert and orientated she sits in her room crying out no screaming "Will somebody help Me please," respectively saying this my ears hear this ringing and in my head I'm thinking does anyone else hear this and my heart crumbles with guilt or sympathy at what cruelty that management has allow to take place. I stop what I'm doing to answer her distress call to find that she just wants to go to the bathroom, and not to urinate on herself.

Two more women sharing a room one pleasantly confused the other diabetic with oxygen and nebulizer treatments. The pleasantly confused patient wears an alarm on the back of her wheelchair along with one on her bed to alarm when she has attempted to transfer without assistance. Her roommate also wheel chair bond alert and orientated very large woman requires a lot of attention as she needs to have her oxygen tank fill, blood glucose levels drawn and nebulizer treatments plus pass her pills, this is a lot for one person. Sometimes instead of getting her blood levels to give insulin I would just fill in a number to have the paperwork look complete. Oh the CNA's where responsible for filling the oxygen tanks and her sometimes didn't get filled so her always had this kind of bluish tint about her lips and fingers.

Another two person room occupied by two women this one shared by one person as the roommate has died in the bed next to her. She too is alert and orientated woman stroke patient with left sided weakness; she is a very heavy set woman requiring a hoer lift to transfer, diabetic and sometimes requires assistance with eating. Brokenhearted she sometimes gets as she remembers her roommates' dying days and all the family member that would come in to set with her, she is crushed as she reminisce about her impending death this went on for many days and she still to this day is troubled. I wondered why, could not this dying woman be moved? To an empty room, to not impose more anguish upon this woman struggling with her on afflictions. You see management is in so much of a hurry to get the rooms occupied there is no room for privacy, for as soon as the bed is empty another person is in it.

The next set of people are some of my favorite one man sleeps on the floor on a mattress due to all his falls the other in a recliner by the window brought from home who never sleeps in the his bed. Both men pleasantly confused but cooperative. The one man that sleeps on the floor by the door has an alarm on the chair and the mattress for moving so if he ends up on the floor it is considered a fall and treated as one, with vital signs and assessment per policy. Also one more treatment order to add to the to do list is checking the wander guard alarms and the fall risk alarms daily to ensure they were working properly. Wander guards are used on the patient's ankle to prevent exiting the facility sounding off the alarm. What happens in the case of the wander guard the patient gets close to the door and the door would sound an alarm and the door would automatically lock, prevent the patient from exiting.

And often times treatment didn't happen, but the blanks were filled in and the more concerning treatments were done according to time. Treatments were sometimes done and other times not depending on the time left prior to going home. Believe me when I say I tried to fit in everything had to be done, and never would seem to finish like the other nurses, until I asked how to get everything done. It was obvious that no matter how long I pressed to get all the work done it wasn't happening so I gave in and starting signing my initials to things I'd hadn't done and just as long as the holes in the book was filled corporate was happy I still had a job and no one was the wiser on how all the work was finished including treatments and any new admissions.

In the hospital the use of restraints was tolerated for the purpose of preventing the patient from causing danger to himself. A nurse could use the wrist restraints at the time needed fill out the necessary paperwork for the doctor and use the restraints for up to 24 hours without a doctor's signature. Why is it not O.K. to use restraint in the long term facilities? If they were allowed some of the deaths cause by falls could be prevented. There was an incident that comes to mind where the patient was in bed at night with restraints improperly applied the patient had somehow slid down to where the restraint was tied across the chest and then to the bed, now the restraint lay across the neck and the patient death resulted from strangulation. What a horrible thing to have happen to this patient every night the patient would have the restraint applied for safety of hurting themselves and very alert patient with some sort of muscular disease that caused involuntary movement, didn't like the restraint but tolerated it just the same because of the safety issues now dead from the very thing that was to keep them safe.

Next a diabetic man, sleeps in the bed next to the door, alert wheels himself in his wheel chair his roommate in a bed next to window a stroke patient that is unable to voice his needs alert, but you would never have guess so. He just stares out in space no expression without blanking eye, on one particular day I had gone in to pass my meds with a glass of supplement drink sometimes given with meds I asked him if he wanted more of the supplement I had given him and he answered by nodding his head. To my surprise he had arrogantly been miss read, for a patient being not alert, and probably for good reason most people assume and never try talking to the patients, because their main objective is to pass the pills and move on. The diabetic man is suppose to receive a night time snack before going to bed but like most things he didn't receive it either because the dietary people don't bring it or the CNA's were too busy, and usually in the early morning this gentleman's blood glucose levels would be dangerous low. Despite all these mishaps the diabetic man is preserved day by day.

The next two are women both somewhat alert the one woman by the door refuses all medicines and eats candy, brought in by her family, instead of her meals no matter how you try to disguise her medicine she will not eat it or drink it in anything. Never drinks much water only sips her urine dark yellow with the dreaded foul smell. Most of the patients' urine was dark and smelly, why because the water was not offered, to those who couldn't reach it on the bedside tables, or the water pitchers weren't filled per shift. The woman by the window intrigues she lays in silence to one side refusing to turn off the side facing the window, now has a pressure sore on the heel of her foot that is blacken and rotting, the smell so horrifying it cuts off your breath. Now she awaits surgery to amputate her foot. Can you only but image how forgotten she must have been, yet she complains only when she is turned has grown accustomed to the pain that she is numb to that side.

Moving to another room two wheelchair bond gentlemen, one by the door has a motorized chair the other by the window a nonmotorized chair. The man by the door a diabetic stroke patient with left sided weakness, noncompliant insulin dependent diabetic eats all kinds of sweets, his family brought in, the doctor orders a sliding scale insulin to cover his high blood glucose levels and for extreme high levels to call for new orders to cover the extreme high ones. Sometimes instead of calling the doctors the blood glucose level would be recorded at the highest on the sliding scale order, as calling the doctor would require time, time that you didn't have. The gentlemen by the window in the nonmotorized chair dies mystery, nothing seem to overly wrong with him but he did complain of his stomach hurting, could it have been an oversight that was missed in his diagnosis or meds not given. He like many others took load of pills daily from early morning till after bedtime at 10 pm.

Next room a qaudpledgic man by the door with a motorized wheel chair lays in bed screams out for help instead of using the call light. This man can use the upper part of his body but not the lower half below the waist. Alert and oriented very needy man likes things just so. Incontinent of bowel and bladder this man bottom looked like someone had taken an ice pick and tried to chip off pieces of his butt. He too didn't get turned or changed often enough, causing excruciating pain when touch to clean him up. A treatment to his bottom was ordered but was never put on accordingly so it got worst till a wound vac had to be put on.

There was a blind man in a semi private room with a roommate, calls to the administration to file a report of abuse. He alleges that he was sexual abuse by a caregiver that had gotten on top of him in the night. This patient alert and oriented, just blind gave details of his attacker that where clear the roommate unable to elaborate was of no help. The caregiver was questioned and advised not to come into contact with this patient again.

Another room a wife separated from her husband due to the availability of men to women roommates. This often happens when insurance is an issue also. This couple married for years now separated but together during meals. Married couples had to be placed in private rooms which were much more expensive than semi-private rooms.

Resident's council meetings were held to hear the voices of the residents' complaints. Most of the complaints came from the more coherent ones. They would say things like the food wasn't prepared properly or some food items they would run out of. Diets weren't being followed so the diabetic people got to eat anything that was served. One man wrote his concerned about emergencies that the staff didn't know what to do, and he was right most of us didn't or didn't feel comfortable about being in an emergency situation.

Resident that can feed themselves or the least likely to be under nutritional guidelines, those who can't feed themselves have nursing assistant help but they get in a hurry having too many patient to assistant will short the patient in eating the meal or leave some patients unfed, the kitchen has it job to do and so they come in to put up trays whether the patient is done or not. Most of the patients suffer great weight loses and the dietician will order ensure drinks to supplement the diet, the nursing assistant knowing this will take the easier way out and give only the ensure drink to rush things along.

In the basement is a locked unit for those suffering from Alzheimer disease so no one can wander off. The risk is still among them their risk of falls and fights, the most forgotten people, all at different levels of memory. The units are set up to accommodate for those with beginning levels of Alzheimer disease, secondary stage, and lastly a unit for those with advance levels of Alzheimer. Each level more difficult than the other the beginning level of memory lost the patient recognize that something is happening to the memory, the second stage the patient clearly unaware of the everyday living necessities like eating sleeping, hygiene, these activities performed with supervision, families are still involved but with much frustration. Last the advance stage almost like zombies without brains wandering around day in day out some seem to not sleep for days, no memory of daily living activities. Most of the medicines given to decrease the advancing of Alzheimer is used in all the patients, but is very difficult to give these medicines to, the nurse will crush the medicines put in the foods the patient is eating to disguise the medicine taste. Some will take it some will not, no one is going to force medicine as some of the Alzheimer patients become very agitated. The nursing assistants become agitated and frustrated with the patient sometimes abuse of the patients is seen or not never the less no reports are made as some patients are fighters. I remember seeing my coworker lead by the hair as a man with Alzheimer grabbed her long ponytail and pulled at it in angra she screamed out while I tried to pry the man's hand off while he swung his other hand at me. This was a very stressful place to say the least frustrating.

The same is true of most long term care facilities across the broad abuse and neglect of patient resident rights, by nursing staff, doctors and agency nurses. Who stands for the patients when management pushes for more performance and little staff to do it? Once I walked in on a management corporate meeting while they sat around the table and talk out how best to use up the entire patient's insurance in what kind of time frame they had to do it. I know the importance of discharge planning but I felt like a thief robbing the poor and needy. What happens when a patient comes in the is half way rehabitable those dollars are used up first even if the time is not yet needed. Say like an injury that needs to heal first prior to intense therapy is performed now the injury is healed and the patient still in need of physical therapy will those dollars are gone and so is the patient to another facility or place that will accept them.

There are other places for the elderly person called retirement homes where many people go to still have some form of independence. Run by companies making large sums of money off the semi will to do people. To be considered for one of these places you must have a large sum of money to just enter the doors had to present thousands of dollars. Yet the company charge the patient for every little item from the necessities like soap and tooth paste, to the needles used to give injections to the mattress pad used on the bed. When I read one of the brochures stating the cost to enter this place I couldn't not believe the amount money that was generated by the corporate heads, yet this pretty place nicely decorated like one of those prize homes featured in the magazines, still had poor management, and poorly staffed. The corporate charged large amounts and promise to cater to the family's wishes of care for the family member. And cater we did, even if the patient needed psychotic medicines, they were not evaluated for them, because the facility was of different levels of assistant living no one who needed total care should have been allowed, but they were and the nursing staff sat around and talked about it. The corporate-heads didn't care at what level the patient was at only that one more facility bed was filled. The staffing suffered with mental abuse from the patient while corporate heads went home. There were many cases that the corporate would promise a certain level of care and didn't have the staff to do it. Once there was several patients admitted to the facility clearly needing evaluation for psych meds distributing other residents yelling out and just having all kinds of behavior but the family refused treatment and the facility honored the family's wishes. It won't be long before someone snips I almost did, I couldn't image one being there day after day, and night after night listening to the out of control patient. The overweight patients that required special equipment to assistant with daily living care or transferring from bed to chair, it simply was not available to use so the standard equipment was used instead. Using the improper equipment caused injuries to both the caregiver and the patient. The patient landed on the floor the employee landed with an injured back or shoulder. Employee injuries are on the raise some of the injuries reported others not, some employees feared losing their jobs. Most of the employees are of ethnic background with no other education other than nursing assistant and that doesn't even require a high school diploma.

Prison nursing is a totally different approach to nursing you see all types of offenders some young trying to be grown but instead just made their 18th birthday still not ready for the world. Now looking at all that foolishness and games they played, they must face the real world of prison. In jail you could see the old and the young men and women whom just started off their young lives in prison for what seem to them as having fun. There were young men imprisoned with some of the nasty wounds that came from these young men running from the police dogs, nurses would see the massive destruction from the dog's gashing teeth marks. Reading some of those men and women history would cause some of the nurses to prejudge and those patients would be treated badly. Take for instead the inmate was in need of pain meds the nurse would purposely make him wait, till she felt like giving it. The prison guards always sided with the nurse and the inmate was always second rated. But for a field of women working in the men's prison was just a rewarding thing some of the nurse would do favors for the inmates. There was a bust of nurses that were caught on camera having and performing sex on the inmates. Some even carried on relationships sending money inside to the inmates and even marrying with them. I have no ill feeling toward inmates as they are people who made mistakes and needed care too, but to some nurses the inmate was either one way or the other.

Agency nurses are more than 50% likely to have mistake pass medication errors occur to the wrong patient and or missing a medication pass or treatment. The error rate triples according to the amount of work per patient that has to be done, as the agency nurse has to be finished according to her allotted time of service render on the contract between the staffing agency and the facility hiring out. The money paid out to the nurse is much more than that of being on a staff position in the hospital or nursing home facility. Agency and staff sometimes don't get along because on staff employees know that agency staffs are getting pay over and above what they are getting paid. I once was considered a DNR or do not return due to a staff who simply did not like me, when I questioned this no one could say why but the agency that I had been going to this place for over a year or so, said they can do what they want. Not fair that hurt my eagle and my pocket book this

DNR had nothing to do with my performance but that one nurse had issues with me call it a personality conflict so you may. This nurse like stewing up trouble saying things like you agency people this and you agency people that. One day after hearing this I spoke up and told her if she felt like we were making so much more money that may she should become agency. She hated agency people coming to this place and talked bad about all of us. We usually got the worst assignments, because we were agency as employee staff member put it "making all that money," and they were correct agency pay was better than being on staff, and they expected agency to work harder for that money.

Staffing agencies also are the backbone to nursing if not for them hospital and Long term care facilities could not survive working short of staff. Agency sometimes use names to fill in shifts that haven't been confirmed to work, then work on filling those shifts at a later time. Many times it has been tried to work short staffed and who suffers non-other than the patient. Hospitals and nursing facilities offer large sign on bonus when staffing is at its all time lowest in manpower. The large sign on bonus that some hospital and nursing homes put in want ads will attract all kinds of nurses good/bad no history checks the only thing that the company is worried about is having a position filled. I went for one of those big sign on bonus once the worst mistake ever. Now I know why companies offer such large sign on bonus, because they are desperate to fill positions where they couldn't keep anyone else to work there for them. Here's how it works you sign a contract between you and the employer to receive the sign on bonus only if agreed upon to work full time and the bonus payable in so many months increments until the last payment in one year. So the company will pay a full time employee set amount of bonus, that is taxable, after 3 months of employment first installment, then 6 months the second installment, the last in one year. Why the staff member couldn't receive the money instead of looking outside for someone new is the million dollars question here the company has let the loyal employee go to hire from outside? Then the new person figures out why the last staff person left it in their head about the big money and so staying doesn't feel so bad the first 3 months and then will for me anyhow the work overcame me and the sign on bonus didn't look so good anymore and I left to keep my sanity.

There are more and more TV programs and sitcoms which paint a picture of perfect sinero scenes of hospitals situations they appear very glamourous and professional for the TV viewer. People aren't interested in the lives of people in the healthcare profession because they see them as these angels on earth, but just like there is a heaven and a hell there're good in bad healthcare professionals. Healthcare is distinguishing profession mostly anyone can identify with being cared for by the nurse and treated by the doctor, but the underlining story is how much do you really know about the people caring for you?.

I am guilty of mistakes and wanting to set the wrong right, it took me some 10 years to confront that which is eating away at my soul. Some mistakes I have done some shared and swore to not tell but to take it to the grave with us. I thank God there were no costly mistakes one resulting in death I just couldn't live with myself. People see me dressed in that nursing uniform and expect you to know everything the truth is I don't everything but I have learned a lot of things in my years of nursing. Family members are the ones most likely to want diagnosis form the nurse in the family instead of going to the doctor for advice, and before you know it you are helping the neighbors, your kids sports team the people at work friends of friends and the list gets longer. I find myself at a nursing burn out ready to explode amazing how involved you are that you lose yourself in the process. Always looking out the welfare of someone else it's easy to lose yourself.

Some time after being a license nurse, I began working for the agency some of them didn't care about the experience that I had, just that my title allow them to fill a shift to make money, no hands on experience. How could the agency put a brand new nurse out in the field without the experience? I tell you it was a scary thing working with patient and passing medications out right out of school. I had given medicine to the wrong patient and even the wrong medicine to the right patient. There was a lot of errors made and know but myself and God know till now. There is not one single nurse that can say they haven't made errors some costly some not so costly.

I was one of the more fortune ones a facility I'd work for, while working as a CNA prior to receiving my license, took me under their wing allow me to shadow one of the staff nurses and pass meds on a few people of 10 until I felt comfortable on my own. What a great feeling of gratitude it was for me having my first nursing experience with people willing to give me a chance, I needed to feel comfortable about this nursing stuff. For more than 7 years I worked as an agency nurse with some good and bad experiences in the Long Term Care Facilities and some Acute Care facilities. And as time went on I became a better nurse handling emergencies and such.

There came the day when a dying man needed my help and the staff nurse knew not what to do I being the agency nurse was suppose to know everything so they say, "agency nurses get the big bucks and know it all," the staff member came to me for help, and I wing through performing CPR on the man while still in his bed until the 911 call was made I didn't have the back broad underlining his body to get a better handle on the chest compressions. I watched as the man took his last breath, the man was dead before the ambulance service got there but the rule is that you can't stop CPR until the emergency team gets there to pronounce the person, so we just went through the motions until that time.

There are good doctors and bad ones too, they make bad mistakes some costly one resulting in death, than malpractice suits pays the patient and all is said and done. The doctor can surrender his license in that state and return to practice in other state. First oath of practice for the doctor is to do no harm some forget to honor this oath. Why these man and woman continue to practice like the other healthcare professional the rule is not to say anything that might hurt or harm the healthcare profession, so most people in this profession know of occurrences and choose to never say anything. Most people fear that by telling you will interfere with a person's livelihood. The number of medication errors is high but there isn't a way of tracking them all or making healthcare professional responsible for these errors. Oh but there is a registry list of nurses whose license are in jeopardy those caught and now facing the State Broad of Health Commission. The list has your name license number the type of offense committed and your nursing status whether you are allowed to practice or awaiting notice.

Is there a nursing shortage you bet there is this career of healthcare is rewarding and stressful. When I asked other nurses about how they felt about the nursing shortage they were quick to answer with yes look how stressful and the pay for being a staff nurse wasn't great, but the job is in demand. More vocational schools are setting up shop and offering degrees in nursing, 18 months for the LPN program and no waiting any entry exam, 24 months for the RN program, some waiting entry exam required.

There is a need for hospitals to go by to being teaching centers for nurses to have hands on experience with a well seasoned nurse in real life situations. There also should be rules for how long of hours a nurse can work and still be physical capable of performing the job effectively, those same rules that apply to the truck drivers. There have been times I would see nurses work more the 5 or 6 days a week 12 hour shifts and make some of the worst mistakes one that directly involved serious injury to the patient. The American people trust the doctors and other healthcare professions to take care of their healthcare needs; never would they suspect anything less than someone professional. My heart goes out to all the nurses who try to do their very best and see all the corruption in this profession and will not say anything to protect this profession. I almost feel like a trader but I'm tired of seeing and knowing and not saying a word. My goal is to be heard and make some changes. God be with each of you healthcare professional remember integrity is not what is seen, rather what you do when you're not seen. One possible solution to the problems with errors is random drug screening and nurses that have the guts to step up and be a part of the solution and stop ignoring it like it isn't about you cause those patients relied on everyone. For those who have been favored to receive much, much is required.

Lightning Source UK Ltd.
Milton Keynes UK
UKOW05f2321111013

218959UK00001B/136/P

9 781607 032373